This Planner Belongs To

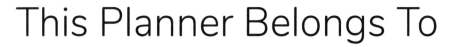

Notes

Notes

CONTACTS

Name	Phone	E-mail @

CONTACTS

Name	Phone	E-mail @

2019

July

	mo	tu	we	th	fr	sa	su
27	1	2	3	4	5	6	7
28	8	9	10	11	12	13	14
29	15	16	17	18	19	20	21
30	22	23	24	25	26	27	28
31	29	30	31	1	2	3	4

August

	mo	tu	we	th	fr	sa	su
31	29	30	31	1	2	3	4
32	5	6	7	8	9	10	11
33	12	13	14	15	16	17	18
34	19	20	21	22	23	24	25
35	26	27	28	29	30	31	1

September

	mo	tu	we	th	fr	sa	su
35	26	27	28	29	30	31	1
36	2	3	4	5	6	7	8
37	9	10	11	12	13	14	15
38	16	17	18	19	20	21	22
39	23	24	25	26	27	28	29
40	30	1	2	3	4	5	6

October

	mo	tu	we	th	fr	sa	su
40	30	1	2	3	4	5	6
41	7	8	9	10	11	12	13
42	14	15	16	17	18	19	20
43	21	22	23	24	25	26	27
44	28	29	30	31	1	2	3

November

	mo	tu	we	th	fr	sa	su
44	28	29	30	31	1	2	3
45	4	5	6	7	8	9	10
46	11	12	13	14	15	16	17
47	18	19	20	21	22	23	24
48	25	26	27	28	29	30	1

December

	mo	tu	we	th	fr	sa	su
48	25	26	27	28	29	30	1
49	2	3	4	5	6	7	8
50	9	10	11	12	13	14	15
51	16	17	18	19	20	21	22
52	23	24	25	26	27	28	29
01	30	31	1	2	3	4	5

2020

January

	mo	tu	we	th	fr	sa	su
01	30	31	1	2	3	4	5
02	6	7	8	9	10	11	12
03	13	14	15	16	17	18	19
04	20	21	22	23	24	25	26
05	27	28	29	30	31	1	2

February

	mo	tu	we	th	fr	sa	su
05	27	28	29	30	31	1	2
06	3	4	5	6	7	8	9
07	10	11	12	13	14	15	16
08	17	18	19	20	21	22	23
09	24	25	26	27	28	29	1

March

	mo	tu	we	th	fr	sa	su
09	24	25	26	27	28	29	1
10	2	3	4	5	6	7	8
11	9	10	11	12	13	14	15
12	16	17	18	19	20	21	22
13	23	24	25	26	27	28	29
14	30	31	1	2	3	4	5

April

	mo	tu	we	th	fr	sa	su
14	30	31	1	2	3	4	5
15	6	7	8	9	10	11	12
16	13	14	15	16	17	18	19
17	20	21	22	23	24	25	26
18	27	28	29	30	1	2	3

May

	mo	tu	we	th	fr	sa	su
18	27	28	29	30	1	2	3
19	4	5	6	7	8	9	10
20	11	12	13	14	15	16	17
21	18	19	20	21	22	23	24
22	25	26	27	28	29	30	31

June

	mo	tu	we	th	fr	sa	su
23	1	2	3	4	5	6	7
24	8	9	10	11	12	13	14
25	15	16	17	18	19	20	21
26	22	23	24	25	26	27	28
27	29	30	1	2	3	4	5

2020

July

	mo	tu	we	th	fr	sa	su
27	29	30	1	2	3	4	5
28	6	7	8	9	10	11	12
29	13	14	15	16	17	18	19
30	20	21	22	23	24	25	26
31	27	28	29	30	31	1	2

August

	mo	tu	we	th	fr	sa	su
31	27	28	29	30	31	1	2
32	3	4	5	6	7	8	9
33	10	11	12	13	14	15	16
34	17	18	19	20	21	22	23
35	24	25	26	27	28	29	30
36	31	1	2	3	4	5	6

September

	mo	tu	we	th	fr	sa	su
36	31	1	2	3	4	5	6
37	7	8	9	10	11	12	13
38	14	15	16	17	18	19	20
39	21	22	23	24	25	26	27
40	28	29	30	1	2	3	4

October

	mo	tu	we	th	fr	sa	su
40	28	29	30	1	2	3	4
41	5	6	7	8	9	10	11
42	12	13	14	15	16	17	18
43	19	20	21	22	23	24	25
44	26	27	28	29	30	31	1

November

	mo	tu	we	th	fr	sa	su
44	26	27	28	29	30	31	1
45	2	3	4	5	6	7	8
46	9	10	11	12	13	14	15
47	16	17	18	19	20	21	22
48	23	24	25	26	27	28	29
49	30	1	2	3	4	5	6

December

	mo	tu	we	th	fr	sa	su
49	30	1	2	3	4	5	6
50	7	8	9	10	11	12	13
51	14	15	16	17	18	19	20
52	21	22	23	24	25	26	27
53	28	29	30	31	1	2	3

July 2019

Sunday	Monday	Tuesday	Wednesday
	1	2	3
7	8	9	10
14	15	16	17
21	22	23	24
28	29	30	31

July 2019

Thursday	Friday	Saturday	Notes
4	5	6	
11	12	13	
18	19	20	
25	26	27	

July

Week 27

○ 1. MONDAY

TO DO

○ 2. TUESDAY

○ 3. WEDNESDAY

NOTES & GOALS

○ 4. THURSDAY

○ 5. FRIDAY

○ 6. SATURDAY / 7. SUNDAY

July

Week 28   07/08/19 to 07/14/19

○ 8. MONDAY

TO DO

_____

_____

○ 9. TUESDAY

_____

_____

_____

_____

○ 10. WEDNESDAY

NOTES & GOALS

_____

○ 11. THURSDAY

_____

_____

_____

○ 12. FRIDAY

_____

_____

_____

○ 13. SATURDAY / 14. SUNDAY

_____

_____

_____

July

○ 15. MONDAY

TO DO

○ 16. TUESDAY

○ 17. WEDNESDAY

NOTES & GOALS

○ 18. THURSDAY

○ 19. FRIDAY

○ 20. SATURDAY / 21. SUNDAY

July

Week 30

○ 22. MONDAY

TO DO

○ 23. TUESDAY

○ 24. WEDNESDAY

NOTES & GOALS

○ 25. THURSDAY

○ 26. FRIDAY

○ 27. SATURDAY / 28. SUNDAY

August 2019

Sunday	Monday	Tuesday	Wednesday
4	5	6	7
11	12	13	14
18	19	20	21
25	26	27	28

August 2019

Thursday	Friday	Saturday	Notes
1	2	3	
8	9	10	
15	16	17	
22	23	24	
29	30	31	

July - August

07/29/19 to 08/04/19

○ 29. MONDAY

TO DO

○ 30. TUESDAY

○ 31. WEDNESDAY

NOTES & GOALS

○ 1. THURSDAY

○ 2. FRIDAY

○ 3. SATURDAY / 4. SUNDAY

August

Week 32   08/05/19 to 08/11/19

○ 5. MONDAY

TO DO

○ 6. TUESDAY

○ 7. WEDNESDAY

NOTES & GOALS

○ 8. THURSDAY

○ 9. FRIDAY

○ 10. SATURDAY / 11. SUNDAY

August

08/12/19 to 08/18/19

○ 12. MONDAY

TO DO

○ 13. TUESDAY

○ 14. WEDNESDAY

NOTES & GOALS

○ 15. THURSDAY

○ 16. FRIDAY

○ 17. SATURDAY / 18. SUNDAY

August

Week 34

08/19/19 to 08/25/19

○ 19. MONDAY

TO DO

○ 20. TUESDAY

○ 21. WEDNESDAY

NOTES & GOALS

○ 22. THURSDAY

○ 23. FRIDAY

○ 24. SATURDAY / 25. SUNDAY

September 2019

Sunday	Monday	Tuesday	Wednesday
1	2	3	4
8	9	10	11
15	16	17	18
22	23	24	25
29	30		

September 2019

Thursday	Friday	Saturday	Notes
5	6	7	
12	13	14	
19	20	21	
26	27	28	

August - September

○ 26. MONDAY

TO DO

○ 27. TUESDAY

○ 28. WEDNESDAY

NOTES & GOALS

○ 29. THURSDAY

○ 30. FRIDAY

○ 31. SATURDAY / 1. SUNDAY

September

Week 36

09/02/19 to 09/08/19

○ 2. MONDAY

TO DO

○ 3. TUESDAY

○ 4. WEDNESDAY

NOTES & GOALS

○ 5. THURSDAY

○ 6. FRIDAY

○ 7. SATURDAY / 8. SUNDAY

September

Week 37

○ 9. MONDAY

TO DO

○ 10. TUESDAY

○ 11. WEDNESDAY

NOTES & GOALS

○ 12. THURSDAY

○ 13. FRIDAY

○ 14. SATURDAY / 15. SUNDAY

September

09/16/19 to 09/22/19

○ 16. MONDAY

TO DO

○ 17. TUESDAY

○ 18. WEDNESDAY

NOTES & GOALS

○ 19. THURSDAY

○ 20. FRIDAY

○ 21. SATURDAY / 22. SUNDAY

September

Week 39

09/23/19 to 09/29/19

◯ 23. MONDAY

TO DO

◯ 24. TUESDAY

◯ 25. WEDNESDAY

NOTES & GOALS

◯ 26. THURSDAY

◯ 27. FRIDAY

◯ 28. SATURDAY / 29. SUNDAY

September - October

○ 30. MONDAY

TO DO

○ 1. TUESDAY

○ 2. WEDNESDAY

NOTES & GOALS

○ 3. THURSDAY

○ 4. FRIDAY

○ 5. SATURDAY / 6. SUNDAY

October 2019

Sunday	Monday	Tuesday	Wednesday
		1	2
6	7	8	9
13	14	15	16
20	21	22	23
27	28	29	30

October 2019

Thursday	Friday	Saturday	Notes
3	4	5	
10	11	12	
17	18	19	
24	25	26	
1			

October

Week 41   10/07/19 to 10/13/19

○ 7. MONDAY

TO DO

○ 8. TUESDAY

○ 9. WEDNESDAY

NOTES & GOALS

○ 10. THURSDAY

○ 11. FRIDAY

○ 12. SATURDAY / 13. SUNDAY

October

10/14/19 to 10/20/19

○ 14. MONDAY

TO DO

○ 15. TUESDAY

○ 16. WEDNESDAY

NOTES & GOALS

○ 17. THURSDAY

○ 18. FRIDAY

○ 19. SATURDAY / 20. SUNDAY

October

10/21/19 to 10/27/19

○ 21. MONDAY

TO DO

_____

....

....

○ 22. TUESDAY

....

....

....

....

○ 23. WEDNESDAY

NOTES & GOALS

_____

....

○ 24. THURSDAY

....

....

_____

_____

○ 25. FRIDAY

_____

_____

_____

_____

_____

○ 26. SATURDAY / 27. SUNDAY

_____

_____

_____

October - November

○ 28. MONDAY

TO DO

○ 29. TUESDAY

○ 30. WEDNESDAY

NOTES & GOALS

○ 31. THURSDAY

○ 1. FRIDAY

○ 2. SATURDAY / 3. SUNDAY

November 2019

Sunday	Monday	Tuesday	Wednesday
3	4	5	6
10	11	12	13
17	18	19	20
24	25	26	27

November 2019

Thursday	Friday	Saturday	Notes
	1	2	
7	8	9	
4	15	16	
1	??	23	
8	29	30	

November

Week 45   11/04/19 to 11/10/19

○ 4. MONDAY

                                           TO DO

○ 5. TUESDAY

○ 6. WEDNESDAY

                                           NOTES & GOALS

○ 7. THURSDAY

○ 8. FRIDAY

○ 9. SATURDAY / 10. SUNDAY

November

11/11/19 to 11/17/19

○ 11. MONDAY

TO DO

○ 12. TUESDAY

○ 13. WEDNESDAY

NOTES & GOALS

○ 14. THURSDAY

○ 15. FRIDAY

○ 16. SATURDAY / 17. SUNDAY

November

11/18/19 to 11/24/19

○ 18. MONDAY

TO DO

○ 19. TUESDAY

○ 20. WEDNESDAY

NOTES & GOALS

○ 21. THURSDAY

○ 22. FRIDAY

○ 23. SATURDAY / 24. SUNDAY

November - December

○ 25. MONDAY

TO DO

○ 26. TUESDAY

○ 27. WEDNESDAY

NOTES & GOALS

○ 28. THURSDAY

○ 29. FRIDAY

○ 30. SATURDAY / 1. SUNDAY

December 2019

Sunday	Monday	Tuesday	Wednesday
1	2	3	4
8	9	10	11
15	16	17	18
22	23	24	25
29	30	31	

December 2019

Thursday	Friday	Saturday	Notes
5	6	7	
12	13	14	
19	20	21	
26	27	28	

December

Week 49

12/02/19 to 12/08/19

○ 2. MONDAY

TO DO

○ 3. TUESDAY

○ 4. WEDNESDAY

NOTES & GOALS

○ 5. THURSDAY

○ 6. FRIDAY

○ 7. SATURDAY / 8. SUNDAY

December

Week 50   12/09/19 to 12/15/19

○ 9. MONDAY

TO DO

○ 10. TUESDAY

○ 11. WEDNESDAY

NOTES & GOALS

○ 12. THURSDAY

○ 13. FRIDAY

○ 14. SATURDAY / 15. SUNDAY

December

12/16/19 to 12/22/19

○ 16. MONDAY

TO DO

○ 17. TUESDAY

○ 18. WEDNESDAY

NOTES & GOALS

○ 19. THURSDAY

○ 20. FRIDAY

○ 21. SATURDAY / 22. SUNDAY

December

12/23/19 to 12/29/19

○ 23. MONDAY

TO DO

○ 24. TUESDAY

○ 25. WEDNESDAY

NOTES & GOALS

○ 26. THURSDAY

○ 27. FRIDAY

○ 28. SATURDAY / 29. SUNDAY

January 2020

Sunday	Monday	Tuesday	Wednesday
			1
5	6	7	8
12	13	14	15
19	20	21	22
26	27	28	29

January 2020

Thursday	Friday	Saturday	Notes
2	3	4	
9	10	11	
16	17	18	
23	24	25	
30	31		

December - January

○ 30. MONDAY

TO DO

○ 31. TUESDAY

○ 1. WEDNESDAY

NOTES & GOALS

○ 2. THURSDAY

○ 3. FRIDAY

○ 4. SATURDAY / 5. SUNDAY

January

○ 6. MONDAY

TO DO

○ 7. TUESDAY

○ 8. WEDNESDAY

NOTES & GOALS

○ 9. THURSDAY

○ 10. FRIDAY

○ 11. SATURDAY / 12. SUNDAY

January

01/13/20 to 01/19/20

○ 13. MONDAY

TO DO

○ 14. TUESDAY

○ 15. WEDNESDAY

NOTES & GOALS

○ 16. THURSDAY

○ 17. FRIDAY

○ 18. SATURDAY / 19. SUNDAY

January

Week 4   01/20/20 to 01/26/20

○ 20. MONDAY

                                         TO DO

○ 21. TUESDAY

○ 22. WEDNESDAY

                                         NOTES & GOALS

○ 23. THURSDAY

○ 24. FRIDAY

○ 25. SATURDAY / 26. SUNDAY

February 2020

Sunday	Monday	Tuesday	Wednesday
2	3	4	5
9	10	11	12
16	17	18	19
23	24	25	26

February 2020

Thursday	Friday	Saturday	Notes
		1	
6	7	8	
3	14	15	
0	21	22	
7	28	29	

January - February

○ 27. MONDAY

TO DO

○ 28. TUESDAY

○ 29. WEDNESDAY

NOTES & GOALS

○ 30. THURSDAY

○ 31. FRIDAY

○ 1. SATURDAY / 2. SUNDAY

February

Week 6

○ 3. MONDAY

TO DO

....
....
....
....
....

○ 4. TUESDAY

○ 5. WEDNESDAY

NOTES & GOALS

....
....
....
....
....

○ 6. THURSDAY

....
....
....

○ 7. FRIDAY

....
....
....
....

○ 8. SATURDAY / 9. SUNDAY

....
....
....

February

Week 7

02/10/20 to 02/16/20

○ 10. MONDAY

TO DO

○ 11. TUESDAY

○ 12. WEDNESDAY

NOTES & GOALS

○ 13. THURSDAY

○ 14. FRIDAY

○ 15. SATURDAY / 16. SUNDAY

February

○ 17. MONDAY

TO DO

○ 18. TUESDAY

○ 19. WEDNESDAY

NOTES & GOALS

○ 20. THURSDAY

○ 21. FRIDAY

○ 22. SATURDAY / 23. SUNDAY

March 2020

Sunday	Monday	Tuesday	Wednesday
1	2	3	4
8	9	10	11
15	16	17	18
22	23	24	25
29	30	31	

March 2020

Thursday	Friday	Saturday	Notes
5	6	7	
12	13	14	
19	20	21	
26	27	28	

February - March

○ 24. MONDAY

TO DO

○ 25. TUESDAY

○ 26. WEDNESDAY

NOTES & GOALS

○ 27. THURSDAY

○ 28. FRIDAY

○ 29. SATURDAY / 1. SUNDAY

March

03/02/20 to 03/08/20

○ 2. MONDAY

TO DO

○ 3. TUESDAY

○ 4. WEDNESDAY

NOTES & GOALS

○ 5. THURSDAY

○ 6. FRIDAY

○ 7. SATURDAY / 8. SUNDAY

March

Week 11   03/09/20 to 03/15/20

○ 9. MONDAY

                                        TO DO

○ 10. TUESDAY

○ 11. WEDNESDAY

                                          NOTES & GOALS

○ 12. THURSDAY

○ 13. FRIDAY

○ 14. SATURDAY / 15. SUNDAY

March

03/16/20 to 03/22/20

○ 16. MONDAY

TO DO

○ 17. TUESDAY

○ 18. WEDNESDAY

NOTES & GOALS

○ 19. THURSDAY

○ 20. FRIDAY

○ 21. SATURDAY / 22. SUNDAY

March

Week 13   03/23/20 to 03/29/20

○ 23. MONDAY

TO DO

○ 24. TUESDAY

○ 25. WEDNESDAY

NOTES & GOALS

○ 26. THURSDAY

○ 27. FRIDAY

○ 28. SATURDAY / 29. SUNDAY

March - April

Week 14   03/30/20 to 04/05/20

○ 30. MONDAY

                               TO DO

○ 31. TUESDAY

○ 1. WEDNESDAY

                               NOTES & GOALS

○ 2. THURSDAY

○ 3. FRIDAY

○ 4. SATURDAY / 5. SUNDAY

April 2020

Sunday	Monday	Tuesday	Wednesday
			1
5	6	7	8
12	13	14	15
19	20	21	22
26	27	28	29

April 2020

Thursday	Friday	Saturday	Notes
2	3	4	
9	10	11	
16	17	18	
23	24	25	
30			

April

Week 15

○ 6. MONDAY

TO DO

○ 7. TUESDAY

○ 8. WEDNESDAY

NOTES & GOALS

○ 9. THURSDAY

○ 10. FRIDAY

○ 11. SATURDAY / 12. SUNDAY

April

○ 13. MONDAY

TO DO

○ 14. TUESDAY

○ 15. WEDNESDAY

NOTES & GOALS

○ 16. THURSDAY

○ 17. FRIDAY

○ 18. SATURDAY / 19. SUNDAY

April

○ 20. MONDAY

TO DO

○ 21. TUESDAY

○ 22. WEDNESDAY

NOTES & GOALS

○ 23. THURSDAY

○ 24. FRIDAY

○ 25. SATURDAY / 26. SUNDAY

April - May

Week 18

○ 27. MONDAY

TO DO

○ 28. TUESDAY

○ 29. WEDNESDAY

NOTES & GOALS

○ 30. THURSDAY

○ 1. FRIDAY

○ 2. SATURDAY / 3. SUNDAY

May 2020

Sunday	Monday	Tuesday	Wednesday
3	4	5	6
10	11	12	13
17	18	19	20
24 / 31	25	26	27

May 2020

Thursday	Friday	Saturday	Notes
	1	2	
	8	9	
4	15	16	
1	22	23	
8	29	30	

May

Week 19

05/04/20 to 05/10/20

○ 4. MONDAY

TO DO

○ 5. TUESDAY

○ 6. WEDNESDAY

NOTES & GOALS

○ 7. THURSDAY

○ 8. FRIDAY

○ 9. SATURDAY / 10. SUNDAY

May

05/11/20 to 05/17/20

○ 11. MONDAY

TO DO

○ 12. TUESDAY

○ 13. WEDNESDAY

NOTES & GOALS

○ 14. THURSDAY

○ 15. FRIDAY

○ 16. SATURDAY / 17. SUNDAY

May

Week 21   05/18/20 to 05/24/20

○ 18. MONDAY

                              TO DO

○ 19. TUESDAY

○ 20. WEDNESDAY

                              NOTES & GOALS

○ 21. THURSDAY

○ 22. FRIDAY

○ 23. SATURDAY / 24. SUNDAY

May

Week 22

05/25/20 to 05/31/20

○ 25. MONDAY

TO DO

○ 26. TUESDAY

○ 27. WEDNESDAY

NOTES & GOALS

○ 28. THURSDAY

○ 29. FRIDAY

○ 30. SATURDAY / 31. SUNDAY

June 2020

Sunday	Monday	Tuesday	Wednesday
	1	2	3
7	8	9	10
14	15	16	17
21	22	23	24
28	29	30	

June 2020

Thursday	Friday	Saturday	Notes
4	5	6	
11	12	13	
18	19	20	
25	26	27	

June

06/01/20 to 06/07/20

○ 1. MONDAY

TO DO

○ 2. TUESDAY

○ 3. WEDNESDAY

NOTES & GOALS

○ 4. THURSDAY

○ 5. FRIDAY

○ 6. SATURDAY / 7. SUNDAY

June

06/08/20 to 06/14/20

○ 8. MONDAY

TO DO

○ 9. TUESDAY

○ 10. WEDNESDAY

NOTES & GOALS

○ 11. THURSDAY

○ 12. FRIDAY

○ 13. SATURDAY / 14. SUNDAY

June

06/15/20 to 06/21/20

○ 15. MONDAY

TO DO

○ 16. TUESDAY

○ 17. WEDNESDAY

NOTES & GOALS

○ 18. THURSDAY

○ 19. FRIDAY

○ 20. SATURDAY / 21. SUNDAY

June

Week 26

06/22/20 to 06/28/20

○ 22. MONDAY

TO DO

○ 23. TUESDAY

○ 24. WEDNESDAY

NOTES & GOALS

○ 25. THURSDAY

○ 26. FRIDAY

○ 27. SATURDAY / 28. SUNDAY

June - July

Week 27

○ 29. MONDAY

TO DO

○ 30. TUESDAY

○ 1. WEDNESDAY

NOTES & GOALS

○ 2. THURSDAY

○ 3. FRIDAY

○ 4. SATURDAY / 5. SUNDAY

Notes

Notes

Notes

Notes

Notes

CONTACTS

Name	Phone	E-mail @

CONTACTS

Name	Phone	E-mail @

Made in the USA
San Bernardino, CA
02 November 2019

59332037R00055